Questions & Answers About Osteoarthritis

Campion Quinn, MD, MHA
Long Island, New York

Larry Greenbaum, MD
Indiana Internal Medicine Consultants
Greenwood, Indiana

JONES AND BARTLETT PUBLISHERS
Sudbury, Massachusetts
BOSTON TORONTO LONDON SINGAPORE

World Headquarters
Jones and Bartlett Publishers
40 Tall Pine Drive
Sudbury, MA 01776
978-443-5000
info@jbpub.com
www.jbpub.com

Jones and Bartlett Publishers
Canada
6339 Ormindale Way
Mississauga, Ontario L5V 1J2
Canada

Jones and Bartlett Publishers
International
Barb House, Barb Mews
London W6 7PA
United Kingdom

Jones and Bartlett's books and products are available through most bookstores and online booksellers. To contact Jones and Bartlett Publishers directly, call 800-832-0034, fax 978-443-8000, or visit our website, www.jbpub.com.

Substantial discounts on bulk quantities of Jones and Bartlett's publications are available to corporations, professional associations, and other qualified organizations. For details and specific discount information, contact the special sales department at Jones and Bartlett via the above contact information or send an email to specialsales@jbpub.com.

Cover Images:
Couple: © Photodisc; *Man:* © Thinkstock; *Woman:* © Ablestock.

ISBN: 978-0-7637-8943-5

The authors, editor, and publisher have made every effort to provide accurate information. However, they are not responsible for errors, omissions, or for any outcomes related to the use of the contents of this book and take no responsibility for the use of the products and procedures described. Treatments and side effects described in this book may not be applicable to all people; likewise, some people may require a dose or experience a side effect that is not described herein. Drugs and medical devices are discussed that may have limited availability controlled by the Food and Drug Administration (FDA) for use only in a research study or clinical trial. Research, clinical practice, and government regulations often change the accepted standard in this field. When consideration is being given to use of any drug in the clinical setting, the healthcare provider or reader is responsible for determining FDA status of the drug, reading the package insert, and reviewing prescribing information for the most up-to-date recommendations on dose, precautions, and contraindications, and determining the appropriate usage for the product. This is especially important in the case of drugs that are new or seldom used.

Production Credits
Executive Publisher: Christopher Davis
Associate Editor: Kathy Richardson
Production Director: Amy Rose
Associate Production Editor: Rachel Rossi
Associate Marketing Manager: Rebecca Wasley
Manufacturing Buyer: Therese Connell
Cover Design: Jon Ayotte
Composition: Appingo
Printing and Binding: Malloy, Inc.
Cover Printing: Malloy, Inc.

Library of Congress Cataloging-in-Publication Data
Quinn, Campion.
100 questions and answers about arthritis / Campion Quinn.
p. cm.
Includes index.
ISBN-13: 978-0-7637-4051-1 (pbk. : alk. paper)
ISBN-10: 0-7637-4051-9
1. Arthritis--Miscellanea. 2. Arthritis--Popular works. I. Title. II. Title: One hundred questions and answers about arthritis.
RC933.Q85 2008
616.7'22--dc22
2007021401

6048

Printed in the United States of America
13 12 11 10 09 10 9 8 7 6 5 4 3 2 1

DEDICATION

This book is dedicated to all those people who suffer from the devastating effects of arthritis and for those doctors who care for them.

CONTENTS

INTRODUCTION

This book was written for people with osteoarthritis and their families. It is the hope of the authors that this book can provide useful information about osteoarthritis and that this information will help the people live healthier and more comfortable lives.

Although this book can be read from cover to cover, it was designed as a reference text, so that an osteoarthritis sufferer or his or her caregiver can review sections whose information is of immediate importance.

This book is not a comprehensive discussion of osteoarthritis. The authors chose to address the questions about this disease that are most frequently asked, in order to explore them in as much detail as possible.

PART ONE

Osteoarthritis: The Basics

What is osteoarthritis?

What causes osteoarthritis?

How does osteoarthritis affect the joints?

More . . .

1. What is osteoarthritis?

Osteoarthritis (OA)

A type of arthritis characterized by pain and stiffness in the joints, such as those in the hands, hips, knees, spine, or feet; it is caused by the breakdown of cartilage.

Osteoarthritis is not an inevitable part of aging. Rather, it is believed to develop in any particular individual as a result of a combination of genetic susceptibility and environmental factors.

Osteoarthritis (OA) is a chronic condition that affects the joints. It occurs more frequently as we age. Of the more than 100 different types of arthritic conditions distinguished, OA is the most common, affecting more than 20 million people in the United States along. It is estimated that if everyone in the U.S. population who is older than age 65 underwent x-rays of their joints, more than half would show evidence of OA in at least one joint. While more than half of the population older than 65 may have OA, however, a large fraction will not. At one time OA was thought to be part of the normal aging process, but we now understand that this disease is not an inevitable part of aging. Rather, OA is believed to develop in any particular individual as a result of a combination of genetic susceptibility and environmental factors.

OA is characterized by inflammation and eventual loss of the cartilage in one or more joints. Cartilage is a complex substance composed of proteins and sugars that serves as a "shock absorber" between the bones of the joints. OA commonly affects the joints of the hands, feet, and spine, as well as the large weight-bearing joints, such as those in the hips and knees.

Symptoms of OA include joint pain, tenderness, decreased range of motion in the affected joints, and a variable amount of swelling and inflammation. OA is a progressive disease, meaning that the symptoms of pain and stiffness tend to worsen over time. The amount of pain and disability that any particular patient will experience is difficult to predict, however. Some patients have OA without symptoms, where the disease is found only incidentally on x-rays. Others have disease that can progress to serious disability and the need for surgery.

The term *osteoarthritis* is derived from a Latin term meaning "joint inflammation." Although the joints affected by OA may exhibit a small amount of inflammation, OA is not considered an inflammatory disease like rheumatoid arthritis (RA). Thus the term OA is technically inaccurate. Some alternative names have therefore been suggested for this condition, including osteoarthrosis, hypertrophic osteoarthritis, and **degenerative joint disease (DJD).**

Degenerative joint disease (DJD)

Joint destruction that occurs over a long period of time. This term is used synonymously with the term "osteoarthritis."

Although it is often referred to as a disease, OA is more appropriately called an arthritic condition that affects one or more joints. This condition results from a variety of disorders that lead to similar symptoms and joint changes. Rheumatologists separate patients with OA into two categories—primary and secondary—based on the cause of the arthritis:

Primary osteoarthritis

The gradual breakdown of cartilage that occurs with age and is caused by stress on a joint.

- Most patients have **primary OA.** Primary OA suggests that the patient has no identifiable predisposing cause for the arthritis.
- Patients with **secondary OA** have an underlying cause for their joint symptoms, such as congenital hip dislocation, major trauma to the joint, joint infection, or a metabolic disease such as hemochromatosis or gout.

Secondary osteoarthritis

Osteoarthritis that results from trauma to the joint or from chronic joint injury due to another type of arthritis, such as rheumatoid arthritis.

Clinically, it is generally not important to make a distinction between the two forms, because their treatment is similar.

2. What causes osteoarthritis?

Despite extensive research, scientists still do not know what causes OA. It is theorized that some type of cartilage damage starts a destructive process that, in genetically susceptible people, results in OA.

While the cause of OA is unknown, many factors are often associated with its development.

Aging

A person's risk for OA increases as he or she gets older, although OA can occur in younger patients, especially those with joint injuries or a history of joint disease (such as hip dysplasia).

Conversely, not every person in their seventies and eighties has OA. OA is not a normal part of the aging process.

Joint Injuries/Wear and Tear

OA occurs early in people who have experienced serious joint trauma, such as football players and ballet dancers. This condition is also encountered more frequently in people who perform heavy labor for a living, as compared to people who work in an office.

Inactivity

The joint cartilage requires frequent compression and relaxation to remain healthy. This activity is believed to help circulate nutrients in the cartilage, which has no vascular supply of its own. People who perform little or no exercise may note that their joints become stiff and painful. This tendency is thought to predispose them to OA.

Obesity

Excess weight puts undue stress on the weight-bearing joints of the body, adding to the wear and tear experienced by the joints. Surprisingly, obese people have an increased incidence of OA in non-weight-bearing joints, such as the fingers and shoulders. Scientists suggest that their fat tissue may release some chemical that predisposes these patients to OA, though this idea is just a theory at this point. Doctors recommend that people with OA try to reach their ideal weight by careful diet and exercise.

Genetics

There appears to be a genetic component to OA. For example, OA of the fingers occurs commonly in families and is most common in women.

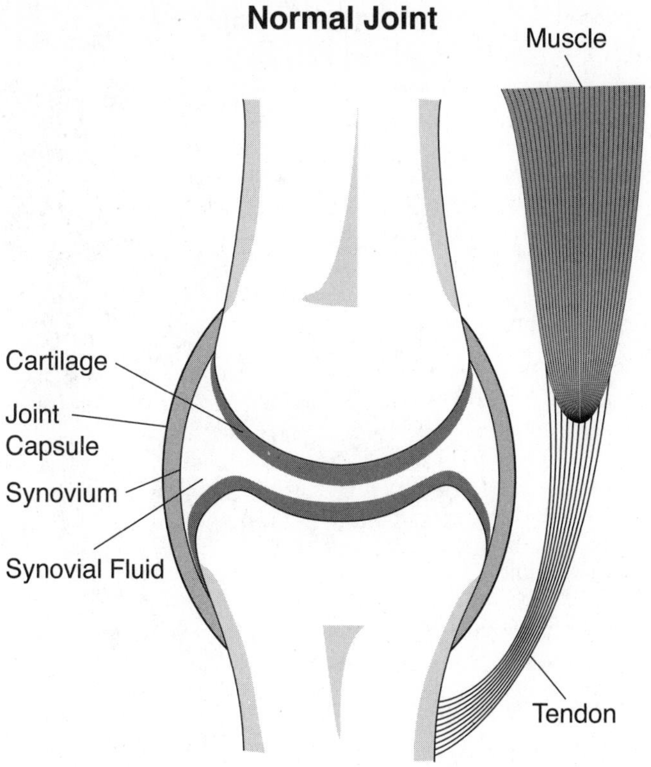

Figure 1 Normal joint.

While the cause of OA remains obscure, people who are at risk for OA, whether because of genetics or occupation, should take care to minimize their chance of developing this condition. To do so, they can participate in regular exercise (preferably low-impact exercise) and pay careful attention to their diet as a means of sustaining an ideal body weight.

3. How does osteoarthritis affect the joints?

OA is a disease of the joints. It predominantly affects the cartilage that lines the bones of the joint (**Figure 1**). Cartilage is the dense rubbery tissue that covers the ends of bones in a joint. In healthy people, its surface is smooth and slippery, which allows the bones in a joint to glide over one another easily. Cartilage also absorbs energy, like a shock absorber,

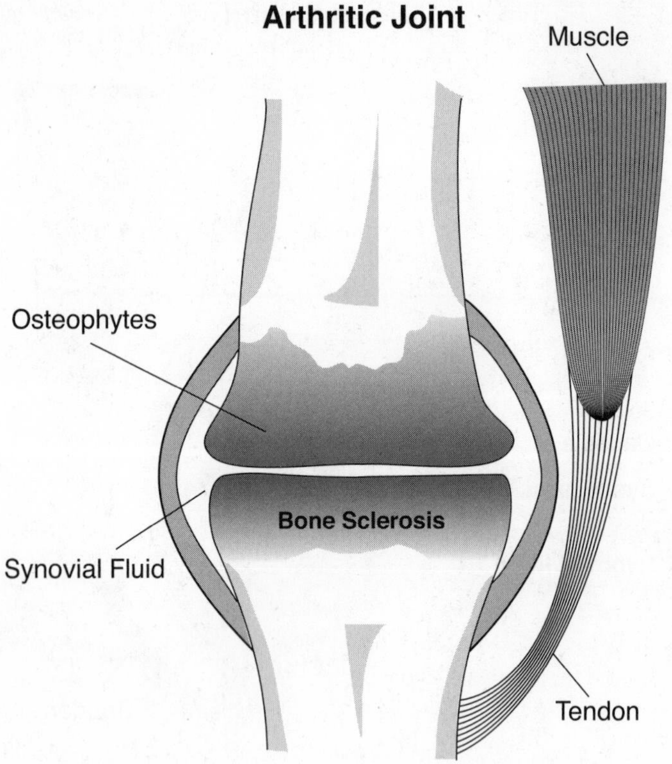

Figure 2 Arthritic joint.

from the jolts associated with movements such as walking. In OA, the cartilage of joints affected becomes inflamed and roughened and wears down. As the disease worsens, the cartilage can disappear completely, so that eventually one bone may rub against the next.

Osteophyte

An outgrowth of bone.

OA affects more than just the cartilage between the bones, however: It also affects the muscles, bones, ligaments and lining of the joint. The bones of the affected joint can undergo many changes. For example, small growths of bone, called **osteophytes** ("bone spurs"), can develop around the joints (**Figure 2**). These bone growths can lead to a knobby appearance and limit the motion of the joint. Small pieces of bone or cartilage may also break off and float inside the joint space, causing pain and further damaging the surface of the cartilage. If a patient has OA of the spine, the bone spurs can press on nerves and cause numbness, tingling, or weakness in the arms or legs.

The bone that underlies the joint is called subchondral bone. In joints affected by OA, subchondral bone can become hardened and brittle and form cysts. In addition, the bone can lose its normal shape, in a process called **bone remodeling.** Scientists believe that subchondral bone remodeling plays an important role in the worsening of symptoms and is a common reason for joint replacements. Some new therapies for OA are aimed at inhibiting bone remodeling. For example, investigators are studying how drugs that are currently employed for the treatment of thinning bones (osteoporosis) will affect patients with OA. These drugs could potentially be used as disease-modifying agents in the treatment of OA.

Bone remodeling

A cyclical process by which bone maintains a dynamic steady state through resorption and formation of a small amount of bone at the same site. Bone remodeling can occur as a result of joint disease.

When a joint affected by OA becomes painful, a person may become reluctant to exercise. As a result, the muscles surrounding the joint can become weak and thin from underuse. Without muscular support, the joint becomes less stable. This instability can lead to misalignment and increased wear on the joint, with resultant pain and disability. This cycle of pain, weakness, and worsening disease can be broken by use of pain medication and adherence to a regular exercise plan. If a painful joint keeps you from the activities you enjoy or from the exercise you need, speak to your doctor. He or she can offer a treatment that may help.

When a joint affected by OA becomes painful, a person may become reluctant to exercise. The resulting cycle of pain, weakness, and worsening disease can be broken, however, by use of pain medication and adherence to a regular exercise plan.

My finger, knee, and thumb joints get very stiff and even more uncomfortable in cool damp weather. Simple things like steering a car, opening bottles, and holding things become bothersome. I find that by using treatments like Tylenol, not carrying things that are heavy (over 5 pounds), and putting my luggage on wheels when traveling helps quite a bit. Also hand massages and warm towels on my hands and fingers help alleviate the discomfort.

—George

4. What is cartilage?

Cartilage is a type of dense connective tissue. It is a tough, semitransparent, flexible tissue that is composed of cartilage cells (**chondrocytes**) and tough fibers that are surrounded by a dense material made of fats and protein (sort of like a fruit salad suspended inside a bowl of Jell-O). Among the many tissues affected by OA, cartilage is the most seriously damaged.

Chondrocyte
A cartilage cell.

In the joints, cartilage covers the surface of the bones and is referred to as **articular cartilage.** A dense fibrous membrane called the perichondrium covers this cartilage. The perichondrium helps to protect the cartilage from wear by allowing one bone to slide over another easily, which reduces friction and prevents damage. Additionally, the thick layer of cartilage found in weight-bearing joints, such as the hips and knees, acts as a shock absorber. In fact, cartilage can resist compressive forces up to 65 times body weight, which also helps to prevent injuries to the bones. Articular cartilage lacks an arterial blood supply and venous and lymphatic drainage. These additional tissues would compromise the cartilage's elasticity and toughness. Given that it does not have its own blood supply, the cartilage derives its nutrition primarily from the surrounding **synovial fluid** and, to a lesser extent, from the blood supply of the adjacent bone. As a consequence of this lack of vasculature, cartilage, once damaged, does not heal readily.

Articular cartilage
Tough, rubbery tissue that forms the surface of bones within joints.

Synovial fluid
A lubricating fluid secreted by the synovial membrane.

Cartilage's toughness and flexibility make it an ideal tissue for lining joints and providing mechanical support to many tissues in the body. For example, it forms part of the structure of the skeleton in the ribs, where it joins them to the breastbone (sternum). Cartilage is found in the tip of the nose, in the external ear, and in the walls of the windpipe (trachea) and the voice box (larynx), where it provides both support and shape. In a human embryo, the entire skeleton is made of cartilage. Even after we are born, many of our bones are little more than cartilage. As we grow and develop, however, these structures absorb calcium and phosphate, causing the bones to become hard and inflexible.

5. What are the risk factors for osteoarthritis?

The cause of OA is elusive in most cases. Nevertheless, physicians have noticed that certain groups have a higher rate of OA than others. You may find that you belong to one or more of these groups.

Age Greater Than 45 Years

Although OA risk increases with increasing age, not all people older than age 45 have degenerating cartilage in their knees and hips. The cartilage in patients with osteoarthritis looks different and has a different chemical composition when compared to "healthy" aged cartilage. Many experts now believe that OA is a disorder caused by a genetic susceptibility combined with injury to the joint. As we grow older, we accumulate more injuries to our joints, our ability to repair injured cartilage decreases, our weight tends to increase, and our chance of developing other forms of arthritis increases.

Female Sex

Women may have some unrecognized factor that predisposes them to accelerated cartilage wear, or perhaps women start out with thinner cartilage plates or have weaker supporting muscles or more lax supporting ligaments. Whatever the cause, women have a higher risk of developing OA. Before age 45, OA occurs more frequently in men; after age 55, it predominantly affects women. In the general population, the ratio of OA in men and women is 3:4.

Hereditary Conditions

Having certain hereditary conditions can predispose you to OA. These conditions include congenital hip dislocation, defective cartilage, and malformed joints. Conditions such as being knock-kneed or being bowlegged also increase the chances for wear and tear in the joint. Additionally, people who have close relatives with OA are at a higher risk for developing it themselves. This increased risk may be the result of a defect in the gene responsible for the formation of **collagen,** which is an important component of cartilage.

Collagen

The major protein of connective tissue, cartilage, and bone.

Ethnicity

The rate of OA is not the same for all ethnic groups. Indeed, both the rate of OA and the distribution of joints affected vary considerably across ethnic groups. In the United States, Caucasian Americans and African Americans have higher rates of OA than Hispanic Americans or members of other ethnic groups. The rate of knee OA in African Americans and Caucasian Americans is about the same, but the rate of OA of the hips is 33% higher in African Americans than in Caucasian Americans. In contrast, Asian Americans have a lower risk of hip OA than Caucasian Americans. Ethnic differences in the rates of OA may be explained by genetic factors that determine the height, weight, joint angles, amount of force, and other structural factors in the joints. Other genes that regulate the chemistry of joint cartilage may also account for these ethnic differences.

History of Joint Injuries

Joint injuries caused by physical activity or sports increases your risk of OA. Football players and ballet dancers, for example, are at higher risk for OA because of the stress that these activities place on their knees and hips. Swimmers and baseball players can suffer from OA of the shoulder or elbow for similar reasons.

Obesity

Obesity, which is defined as being 20% over one's healthy weight, is a known risk factor for OA. Being obese dramatically increases the stress on weight-bearing joints and accelerates degeneration once OA has started. Obese people commonly develop OA of the hips and knees, but they also have a higher risk of developing OA of the fingers. Some scientists have suggested that excess fat tissue causes increased cartilage inflammation even in non-weight-bearing joints.

Other Arthritis

People who have another disease that affects the joints are at a higher risk for developing OA. Diseases such as rheumatoid arthritis, hemochromatosis, gout, and pseudogout, for example, can change the normal structure and function of cartilage and lead to early degeneration.

Education

As unlikely as it sounds, your level of education is associated with your risk of OA. Medical studies have found that the incidence of OA is highest in people with lower educational levels. One study, completed in 2000, demonstrated that college graduates had half the rate of OA as compared to those people who didn't graduate from high school. It is unlikely that reading and studying somehow make your joints healthier. Instead, college graduates may merely represent a different population of people from those without a high school diploma. College graduates, as a group, may have different ethnic backgrounds, have a lower ratio of women to men, and be less likely to be engaged in occupations that require physical labor as compared to people who didn't graduate from high school.

6. What is the prognosis for osteoarthritis?

In a worst-case scenario, a joint affected by OA can become stiff and painful. These symptoms result from the loss of the smooth, gliding surface that undamaged cartilage provides. As the disease progresses, the cartilage in a joint becomes thin and ragged, and more stiffness and a "catching" sensation may occur. These problems may cause a person to restrict the motion of that joint, which can in turn cause the surrounding ligaments to contract and tighten. The muscles that move the joint may ultimately become weakened and thin, with the overall effect being a loss of mobility and a disruption of work and recreation. This is a dire prediction, but not an unavoidable one: It reflects a scenario where the person with OA receives no medical care.

The prognosis for osteoarthritis is generally very good.

In reality, the prognosis for OA is generally very good. Many people ask, "Isn't rheumatoid arthritis the crippling arthritis—the type of arthritis that leads to disability?'" This question suggests that the prognosis for rheumatoid arthritis (RA) is bad, and the prognosis for all other types of arthritis is much better. This is an oversimplification. It is possible to have a mild case of RA or a severe case of OA. Moreover, many factors affecting the final outcome of arthritis depend on the person seeking treatment. Specifically, is the individual compliant with that treatment prescribed, is he or she receiving timely medical care, and does the individual work to maintain a healthy lifestyle?

It is difficult to predict the outcome of OA based on a history and physical exam. One person may have a relatively mild course of OA affecting a few joints; another may develop severe disease in many joints that render him or her unable to work. Some new studies suggest that "active synovitis" or inflammation of the cartilage seen on magnetic resonance imaging (MRI) or bone scan suggests a more aggressive and debilitating course of disease, although the results of these studies are still being debated. Some risk factors suggestive of a more disabling course of OA are believed to include obesity, early age of disease onset, sedentary lifestyle, traumatic joint injuries, and joint x-rays that show very little joint space or "bone-on-bone" contact between the bones of the joint.

Predicting the severity of anyone's OA is difficult. Nevertheless, identifying risk factors for progression of disease gives doctors and patients an opportunity to improve those risks that can be modified.

7. Is osteoarthritis an inherited disease?

Specialists in arthritic disease are often asked if OA is an inherited disease. People with OA are concerned about the possibility of their siblings developing the same problem or about their chances of "passing" the disease to their children.

Studies of large populations of patients have demonstrated that OA does, indeed, have a major genetic component. Researchers have found that a pattern of heritability exists among joint sites. That is, if a parent has OA of the hip, there is a higher likelihood of his or her child having OA of the hip. Similar patterns have been identified for knee and spine OA. Unfortunately, the results across many studies are not always consistent. These discrepancies may arise because different investigators perform these studies a little differently. For example, they may use different populations of patients (older, younger, different ethnicities, and so on), different definitions of disease, and different ways of interpreting physical exams and x-rays. This complicates the task of understanding the complex genetics underlying OA.

Advances in DNA mapping have led arthritis specialists to examine the genetic makeup of individuals with OA to see if it differs from the genetic makeup of people without OA. Researchers in Asia have already identified variations in a gene responsible for the development of cartilage that is associated with a higher risk of hip and knee OA in Japanese and Chinese patients. This gene, which is called GDF5, was found to be more common in patients with OA than in a similar-size group of people without OA. These findings do not imply that GDF5 is the only gene that affects OA, however. The variations of the incidence of disease in populations affected, in the distribution of joints affected, and the inheritance pattern of this disease suggest that more than one gene may be involved and that other environmental factors may influence the onset and progression of OA.

To get a better understanding of the genetics of OA, an international research network has launched the largest study ever in an attempt to discover the source of the genetic susceptibility for OA. Scientists in the United States and the United Kingdom are studying families of people with OA. After taking detailed histories of patients, their family history of OA, and their risk factors for OA, these researchers will perform a complete physical exam of each patient, including x-rays of the hand, hip, knee, and lower spine. Next, blood samples will be taken for DNA testing. The researchers will then analyze the DNA samples and x-rays and chart the family tree in an attempt to identify the genes involved. If this study succeeds in pinpointing the gene or group of genes that cause OA, doctors may be able to identify those patients who are at risk for OA early and help them modify their lifestyles to slow the onset and reduce the symptoms of the disease. In the future, perhaps an effective treatment or a cure can be found with more modern genetic techniques.

Today, however, you should inform your doctor of any family history of OA. This information should include how the affected family members are related to you, which joints were affected, and how they were treated. For example, did that family member use a cane, take any specific medications, or have a joint replacement? This information will give your physician a better idea of your own risk for developing OA, including which joints may be affected and which risk factors you might be able to modify so as to reduce the impact of this disease.

8. What are the symptoms of osteoarthritis?

OA is principally a disease of the joints. As a consequence, its symptoms include pain, swelling, and stiffness of the joints.

The pain associated with OA usually has an insidious onset, is generally described as aching or throbbing, and may result from changes that have occurred over the last 15 to

20 years. It is usually worsened by activity and improved by rest. As the disease progresses and the joint becomes more damaged, the pain may become constant. This pain does not come from an irritation of the cartilage (which contains no nerves), but rather from the adjacent tissues that are stretched or inflamed.

Joint stiffness is another cardinal finding in OA. Morning stiffness can be found in all types of arthritis. This stiffness usually lasts about 30 minutes with OA, compared to an hour or more for rheumatoid arthritis. Many people with OA notice that their joints become stiff after they remain in the same position for long periods of time, such as after sitting or driving. Doctors sometimes call this type of stiffness "gelling." A few minutes of movement typically dispels this type of stiffness. The symptoms of stiffness can be improved by taking nonsteroidal anti-inflammatory drugs (NSAIDs), such as ibuprofen or indocin, or by taking a hot shower or bath.

Swelling of the joints is another classic feature of OA. It is caused by changes in the bone and fluid in the joint. The progressive destruction of the cartilage "cushion" leads to the release of chemicals that affect the bones of the joint. The ends of the bones can enlarge and form bony growths (bone spurs). These growths increase the appearance of joint enlargement or "knobbiness." An increase in the amount of joint fluid present also contributes to joint swelling. The erosion of cartilage results in an inflammation of the lining of the joint (called the **synovial membrane**). The synovial membrane produces excess fluid that collects in the joint, and this fluid production can increase with increased exercise or joint injury. As this fluid buildup can cause increased pressure and pain, doctors sometimes remove it to relieve symptoms.

Synovial membrane

Connective tissue that lines the cavity of a joint and produces synovial fluid.

OA typically affects the joints of the hand—principally the middle knuckle joints, the distal knuckle joints (next to the fingernail), and the base of the thumb. The hips, knees, feet (especially the big toe), neck, and low back are other com-

Heberden's nodes

Knobby overgrowths of the joint nearest the fingertips in patients with osteoarthritis.

mon sites for OA. Finger joints affected by OA exhibit a hard bony swelling called **Heberden's nodes.** Sometimes early in the course of the disease there may be redness around the affected joint, similar to that seen with rheumatoid arthritis. Your doctor can usually tell the two types of arthritis apart, even without taking x-rays. In more advanced cases of OA, patients may experience a decreased range of motion in the affected joints.

Arthritis of the hip or knee affects a person's ability to get up or down from a seated position as a result of pain and stiffness. The change from sitting to standing puts more weight on your hips and knees than walking or standing; thus, the lower the seat, the harder it becomes to stand up. Many people describe great difficulty getting up, but after they are up they can walk. Purchasing chairs with higher seats and arm rests can help overcome this difficulty.

When OA strikes the spine, it can lead to pain and stiffness in the neck or low back. People with spinal OA complain of pain when they turn their heads or touch their toes. In addition, advanced spinal OA can produce bone spurs along the vertebrae. These bone spurs can pinch nerves along the spine, resulting in numbness and tingling of the hands or feet.

Secondary (indirect) problems created by OA include anxiety or depression, feelings of helplessness or dependence on others, and decreased ability to perform activities of daily living or work.

PART TWO

Diagnosing Osteoarthritis

How does a doctor make the diagnosis of osteoarthritis?

Are bumps on the fingers a sign of osteoarthritis?

Does my doctor need to do x-rays to diagnose osteoarthritis?

More . . .

9. How does a doctor make the diagnosis of osteoarthritis?

Your doctor makes the diagnosis of OA on the basis of your history and the results of your physical examination. People with OA usually complain of pain, stiffness, or joint swelling, or some combination of these symptoms. During your physical exam, your doctor will pay special attention to your joints. He or she will check for swelling, tenderness, redness, joint effusions (fluid inside the joint), and your ability to flex and extend the affected joints. Your physician will also evaluate the distribution of affected joints. The pattern of distribution of inflamed joints varies according to the type of arthritis and can be an important clue in making a diagnosis of OA. For example, OA typically affects the middle knuckle joints, the distal knuckle joints (next to the fingernails), and the base of the thumb. The hips, knees, feet (especially the big toe), neck, and low back are other common sites for OA. In comparison, rheumatoid arthritis (RA) typically affects the wrists and the first knuckle joints of the hands; these joints are seldom affected by OA. Your doctor should look for other physical findings associated with OA, such as muscle wasting and weakness.

The diagnosis of osteoarthritis is made on the basis of your history and the results of your physical examination. There is no particular test whose results can be used to make a definitive diagnosis of OA.

There is no particular test whose results can be used to make a definitive diagnosis of OA, so special tests such as blood tests and x-rays are usually not needed when this condition is suspected. Occasionally, your doctor may order one or more of these tests if he or she needs to exclude other arthritic conditions. Blood tests and radiographs may also be helpful for monitoring for side effects of medications or to help determine the extent of joint damage when considering surgical treatment.

10. Are bumps on the fingers a sign of osteoarthritis?

People with OA can develop swelling and redness around the joints of their fingers. Bumps around the farthest joints in your fingers (the ones farthest from your wrist) are called Heberden's nodes. They are typically about the size of a pea and are sometimes painful when they first develop, but frequently become less painful later. These knobby bumps are named after a British doctor, William Heberden, who worked in London at the time of the American Revolution.

Bouchard's nodes

Knobby overgrowths of the middle joint of the fingers in people with osteoarthritis.

Bumps around the next set of finger joints (the joints in the middle of the fingers) are called **Bouchard's nodes.** These nodes were first described by a French physician, Charles Joseph Bouchard, who worked in Paris during the nineteenth century. Bouchard's nodes occur less commonly than Heberden's nodes. Both types of nodes are caused by the same inflammatory process that causes swelling and pain in the hips and knees, and both are classic signs of OA.

Bouchard's and Heberden's nodes usually develop during middle age and begin with swelling and redness. The swelling is at first painful and tender; later, the redness goes away, and the pain and tenderness become less pronounced. The swelling is caused by inflammation of the cartilage in the finger joint. Eventually, small amounts of bone grow around the joint, leading to bone spurs. The nodes become hard and immovable. Infrequently, the nodes can become large enough to cause numbness in the fingertips and make it difficult to flex the fingers or make a fist. They may even cause the fingers to deviate sideways.

Heberden's nodes are more commonly found in women than in men. These nodes rarely require treatment, but if they reduce the functioning of the hand, surgery can help.

11. Does my doctor need to do x-rays to diagnose osteoarthritis?

When a person presents to a physician with complaints of joint pain and swelling, the doctor understands that numerous conditions could cause these symptoms. The history you provide and the results of your physical exam may point to one or more diagnoses. It is helpful to have further evidence to help clarify one diagnosis and eliminate others. Therefore, it is appropriate to perform x-rays on any swollen and painful joint to help determine the cause of these symptoms.

People with OA have characteristic changes in the joints that can be seen on an x-ray. These changes include an uneven loss of cartilage in the joint, called "loss of joint space" on the x-ray interpretation. Small growths of bone (bone spurs) may develop around the joints, and the bone underneath the cartilage may become thickened or hardened (bony sclerosis). In addition, the bone may change shape and develop cysts. In the early stages of OA, these bone changes may appear on x-rays, but the patient may not experience any pain or swelling.

Although x-rays cannot conclusively confirm the presence of OA, they can be a useful tool for distinguishing between OA and rheumatoid arthritis, gout, and other conditions. Additionally, x-rays establish a baseline for comparison. As the disease progresses, they can be used to monitor changes in the bones over time. Often, as part of a person's initial evaluation with a rheumatologist, chest x-rays are ordered in addition to x-rays of any swollen joints. Chest x-rays are performed to evaluate the lungs for diseases that are sometimes associated with arthritis.

X-rays are usually performed in a special hospital department (Radiology) by a radiologic technician or a radiographer, who will tell you which part of your body is to be x-rayed. These technicians are highly skilled. They must have college degrees, undergo additional training, and pass a state licensing examination before they can take x-rays. These technician's training is different from that of the radiologist—a radiologist is a physician who is trained to interpret x-ray images.

To make the image, x-rays are passed through your body and captured on special film. This film is then developed and examined. Standard x-rays are particularly good at showing abnormalities of the bone, but they rarely show problems in soft tissues. For this reason, they do not show the changes associated with early-stage arthritis very well. Despite this drawback, x-rays can highlight areas that help the doctor to diagnose arthritis, such as damaged areas on the bone.

I am not certain about diagnosis not concerning the spine. In my case MRI's were performed to confirm the diagnoses and pinpoint the areas in the neck and spine that were causing the pain.

—George

Learning more about your own disease will help you better understand why your doctor recommends certain treatments and asks you to avoid others. It will also help you feel in control of your osteoarthritis and lead you to become an active participant in your own care.

12. Is it important to learn more about my osteoarthritis?

While you don't have to get a medical degree, learning more about your own disease will help you better understand why your doctor recommends certain treatments and asks you to avoid others. In addition, knowing more about your disease will help you feel in control of your OA and lead you to become an active participant in your own care.

There are many things that you can learn about OA, such as how it starts, what makes it worse, and what can help to reduce joint pain and impairment. In one study of adults who were provided with a self-help educational program, doctors found that even four years later, those patients who had completed the educational program had more knowledge of OA, had less joint pain, and tended to comply more with recommended therapies, compared with similar patients who didn't participate in the educational program.

The Arthritis Foundation sponsors an arthritis self-help course, which is intended to teach people with OA about the latest pain management techniques, the newest medications, and the best ways to manage stress and fatigue. You can learn more about this program by calling your local chapter of the Arthritis Foundation or going on the Internet and looking at the following website: http://www.arthritis.org/events/getinvolved/ProgramsServices/ArthritisSelfHelp.asp.

It is most definitely important to learn more. This is a progressive disease; we need to understand how this works, what to expect, how to deal and live with it. It is also extremely important to understand that new treatments and drugs are constantly being utilized. The more you learn the better you will be able to manage it and enjoy life.

—George

PART THREE

Treatment of Osteoarthritis

What are some medical treatments for osteoarthritis?

What are nondrug treatments for osteoarthritis-related pain?

Can a change in diet improve or reverse osteoarthritis?

More . . .

13. What are some medical treatments for osteoarthritis?

Osteoarthritis is the most common type of arthritis. Although it cannot be cured, its symptoms—such as pain, stiffness, and swelling—can usually be managed effectively. Doctors try to achieve this goal with the least amount of medication possible and with the safest medications possible.

Regular exercise is very helpful in relieving symptoms and preventing disease progression; maintaining a normal body weight is also important.

Regular exercise is very helpful in relieving symptoms and preventing disease progression; maintaining a normal body weight is also important in this regard. Aerobic exercise and exercises to strengthen the quadriceps (a large muscle in the front of the thigh) are particularly helpful for treating OA of the knee or hip.

Likewise, walking aids such as canes are helpful in the management of hip and knee OA. These devices decrease pain by reducing the weight placed on an arthritic hip or knee. Their use allows for increased physical activity.

If you use a cane, you should hold it in the hand opposite the knee or hip that is hurting. For example, if your right knee hurts, hold the cane in your left hand. Some people associate the use of a cane with age and disability. Those people may choose to use a cane selectively—for example, when they know they will be walking some distance, as in a fairground or shopping mall. Using the cane this way can alleviate flare ups of discomfort both during and after the activity.

Taping of the patella can be helpful for relieving some types of knee pain. A wide variety of different knee braces can also be very helpful in such cases. A physical therapist can assist you in deciding whether any of these treatments are right for you. Many of these treatments have been discussed elsewhere in this book as well.

If medication is necessary, then the safest drugs should be selected first. Many people will do well taking acetaminophen (brand name: Tylenol). Although this drug is not an anti-inflammatory medication, for many people it is an effective treatment for pain. Unlike many prescription medications, acetaminophen is inexpensive, readily available, and relatively safe. The side effects most commonly associated with acetaminophen include nausea, constipation, and occasionally drowsiness. The most worrisome side effect is liver toxicity, though this problem is exceedingly rare when acetaminophen is taken as directed.

If acetaminophen doesn't work or doesn't work well enough, a nonsteroidal anti-inflammatory drug (NSAID) can be tried. These medications are available both in over-the-counter formulations and in higher doses by prescription from your doctor. The side effects most commonly encountered with this class of medication are upset stomach and ulcer complications. The risk of stomach ulcers is greatest in those individuals who have acid reflux disease, use corticosteroids, smoke tobacco, or drink alcohol. Those persons who are at highest risk for ulcer disease may need to take additional medications such as cimetidine (Tagamet) or omeprazole (Prilosec) to help protect their stomachs against these side effects. Misoprostol (Cytotec) can also be used to protect the stomach, but it produces upset stomach symptoms as well, so it is not used frequently for this purpose. Unfortunately, the need to protect the stomach increases the number of pills that must be taken—and hence the cost of treatment.

Taking NSAIDs is also associated with a risk of damage to your kidneys. This risk is greatest in people who are older than 65, individuals with hypertension or congestive heart failure, or those taking diuretics or angiotensin-converting enzyme (ACE) inhibitors. Patients who are on anticoagulation therapy, such as those taking warfarin (Coumadin) or heparin, should also use NSAIDs with caution.

Members of a newer type of NSAID class, called COX-2 inhibitors (such as Celebrex), have received a lot of attention recently. These medications have a little less risk of serious stomach complications such as ulcers, but they are much more expensive than the older NSAIDs, and their safety advantage for the stomach is cancelled out if you take even a small dose of aspirin. Two other COX-2 inhibitors, named Vioxx and Bextra, were removed from the market because they were associated with an increased risk of heart disease. For these reasons, this type of medication offers only a small advantage for a limited number of people with OA.

Older NSAIDs called nonacetylated salicylates (e.g., salsalate, trilisate) are a good choice for some people, especially those who have experienced stomach upset with other NSAIDs or those who have decreased kidney function. These medications are relatives of aspirin, although they are chemically different than regular aspirin. Nonacetylated salicylates are inexpensive and are less likely to cause upset stomach or kidney problems than many other NSAIDs. They can cause ringing in the ears, difficulty hearing, or dizziness if their levels in the blood become too high, but these side effects disappear quickly if the medication is temporarily stopped.

If you are taking a narcotic painkiller on a regular basis, it is appropriate to be under the care of a pain specialist. A pain specialist can help to maximize your pain relief while avoiding the side effects and dependency linked to these medications.

Many people with OA are intolerant of the side effects of NSAIDs or still have pain despite treatment with these drugs. For these people, physicians may prescribe narcotic pain medications, such as codeine, morphine, or synthetic morphine derivatives (e.g., hydrocodone, oxycodone). These medications have no anti-inflammatory effects but can treat pain very effectively. They are unlikely to cause ulcers, but can cause upset stomach, drowsiness, constipation, or other side effects. Some people believe that there is a stigma attached to taking pain medications, and many worry—unnecessarily—about becoming "addicted" to pain medication. If you are taking a narcotic painkiller on a regular basis, it is appropriate to be under the care of a pain specialist. A pain specialist can help to maximize your pain relief while avoiding the side effects and dependency linked to these medications.

Marijuana has a long history of medicinal use. For millennia, many cultures have used preparations of this herb to treat pain. In the United States, marijuana was widely used for this purpose as late as the 1800s. Several studies have found that marijuana does, indeed, have analgesic effects. In fact, the active ingredient in marijuana, called tetrahydrocannabinol (THC), may work as well in treating cancer pain as the narcotic medication codeine. When given to patients taking opiate pain medications, marijuana seems to enhance the pain relief associated with those medications, which could allow for the use of lower doses of opiate pain relievers in patients suffering from chronic pain. Scientists and pain specialists are currently developing new medications based on marijuana to treat pain.

To be clear, marijuana is an illegal substance in the United States. In June 2005, the U.S. Supreme Court ruled, in a 6-3 decision, that people whose doctors have prescribed marijuana for medical purposes can be arrested and prosecuted, overriding medicinal marijuana statutes in ten states. In their decision, the members of the Court emphasized that their ruling was not based on whether marijuana is effective for pain relief.

Corticosteroid injections can be very helpful in OA. **Viscosupplementation** injections (e.g., Hyalgan, Synvisc) can relieve knee pain if nothing else works. In viscosupplementation, a rheumatologist or orthopedic surgeon use hyaluronic acid injections to treat the knees of people affected with OA. The addition of this hyaluronic acid to the joints provides a cushioning and lubricating effect. In addition, hyaluronic acid injections provide pain relief even after medication is no longer detectable in the joint. These injections are an alternative to corticosteroid injections for people with knee pain that is not manageable with physical therapy and pills. When pain is constant and medications and other conservative treatments

Viscosupplementation

A treatment option for people with osteoarthritis of the knee that involves the injection of hyaluronan, a natural component of synovial fluid, directly into the knee joint.

offer little relief, surgical treatment should be considered. Pain and limited mobility should not be accepted as "part of the disease process." Discuss your pain with your doctor, and seek out the best therapy together.

I have had some good results from acupuncture in the early stages. Also I found massages of the hands and feet help, as well as hot wax treatment for my hands and fingers.

—George

14. What are nondrug treatments for osteoarthritis-related pain?

Pain can be the predominant symptom in OA, and it is a major cause of the disability associated with this type of arthritis. Your doctor should assess the level of pain that you have at each meeting and determine how much this pain is affecting your ability to function. This assessment provides a rational basis for a pain treatment program. Your doctor should teach you about pain, pain management options, and self-management programs as part of any OA treatment plan.

OA pain is traditionally treated with nonsteroidal anti-inflammatory drugs (e.g., ibuprofen, naproxen) if it is of moderate intensity, or with medications from the opiate family (e.g., demerol, morphine, hydrocodone) if it is severe. But what if these medications are not controlling the pain and surgery is not an option? What other options are available?

Experts in pain management recognize that pain is not simply the result of a physical problem, but has psychological and social dimensions, too. Addressing all of these areas is important when treating pain.

A group of therapies, collectively known as cognitive-behavioral therapy (CBT), addresses the physiologic, psychological, and social dimensions of pain. In fact, current research supports the use of CBT as an effective means to reduce pain and improve function in OA. CBT is based on the idea that thought and behavior patterns can worsen the perception of pain and contribute to feelings of helplessness and fatigue. These feelings can be significant obstacles to recovery. The goal of CBT, then, is to alter the way you think and behave when you feel pain. CBT is not a single treatment, but rather a group of treatments, each of which employs a different modality to reduce pain—for example, stress management, relaxation techniques, and cognitive restructuring.

Both anxiety and stress have negative effects on patients with OA. Pain and its accompanying disability can increase a person's stress level. Conversely, stresses from work, family, or the environment can increase a person's perception of pain. Stress management is used to break this cycle of stress and pain and minimize a patient's response to stress. First, you learn to recognize those situations or occurrences that trigger stress. Once identified, you can learn to avoid these stressful conditions. When avoidance isn't possible, relaxation training may provide relief. Relaxation training can take the form of biofeedback, progressive relaxation exercises, or guided imagery. All of these techniques can reduce muscle tension, which can in turn aggravate pain, and allow you a chance to shift your attention away from your pain, which reduces your perception of pain.

Negative thoughts that are associated with pain are often erroneous and distorted, but can nevertheless worsen your pain and increase your emotional distress. Cognitive restructuring is a technique that attempts to deal with this problem. Patients are taught to identify the negative thoughts that enter the mind when they experience pain. For example, you might think, "This pain is the worst I've ever felt. I'll never get better. Maybe there's something else the matter with me, like cancer." A therapist can help you first challenge the validity of these thoughts and then modify them. For example, you might tell yourself, "I've had this kind of pain before and got better in a few hours" or "This pain is bad, but I haven't had a flare in a month since starting my exercise program. I'm really getting better."

Cognitive-behavioral therapy is an important and effective therapy that can reduce pain and psychological disability and enhance a person's self-efficacy and pain coping skills. It should be integrated with other treatments in a multi-disciplinary approach to the treatment of osteoarthritis.

CBT is an important and effective therapy that can reduce pain and psychological disability and enhance a person's self-efficacy and pain coping skills. This does not imply that you should replace all of the more common pain treatments with CBT, but rather that this technique should be integrated with other treatments in a multidisciplinary approach to the treatment of OA.

15. Can a change in diet improve or reverse osteoarthritis?

Many claims are made that changes in diet can prevent, improve, or reverse the symptoms of OA. These diets suggest eliminating your consumption of red meats, "acidic" foods (such as tomatoes and peppers), fatty foods (red meat and dairy products), processed sugar, or alcohol. Proponents of these diets contend that these substances cause "allergies" or other immune reactions, which are manifested as OA. Other diets recommend adding certain foods to treat OA, such as fish oils, green vegetables, seaweed, seeds, and whole grains. These foods are thought to contain micronutrients, antioxidants, and other substances that will prevent the onset of OA. Still other diets promote regular fasting as a way of "cleansing the body" and decreasing the amount of immunological irritants one takes in.

Currently, medical research does not support the concept that modifying your diet or eating larger amounts of certain foods will prevent OA or reverse its effects. Additionally, the regular consumption of "acidic" foods is not associated with an increased risk of OA. While the use of moderate amounts of alcohol and tobacco are not recommended as a general rule, their consumption has not been associated with increased rates of OA.

Despite these facts, diet is an important part of a healthy lifestyle, and research suggests that some changes in diet may be helpful when you have OA. Specifically, the goals of a healthy diet in individuals with OA should be to treat obesity and osteoporosis.

Diet is an important part of a healthy lifestyle. The goals of a healthy diet in individuals with osteoarthritis should be to treat obesity and osteoporosis.

Overweight persons might reduce their chances for developing or aggravating their osteoarthritis by losing weight. Obesity increases the risks associated with most types of surgery and makes rehabilitation following orthopedic surgery more difficult. Furthermore, if a person already has osteoarthritis in a weight-bearing joint, having a higher body weight can accelerate the joint damage. Therefore, a diet low in calories can ameliorate at least this risk factor.

The principal mineral in bones is calcium; vitamin D is necessary for the body to absorb and use calcium. People with low calcium and vitamin D intakes can suffer from osteoporosis, which is itself a risk factor for OA. Specialists in the treatment of osteoporosis recommend exercise and adequate calcium intake, as recommended for age and gender, to help maintain bone density. In addition, supplementation with vitamin D can help prevent bone loss. In particular, vitamin D deficiency has been shown to increase a person's risk for OA disease progression. Although supplementation of vitamin D in patients with normal vitamin D levels has not been shown to decrease the rate of OA progression, taking the recommended daily requirement of this vitamin is not associated with adverse events.

16. Can losing weight improve my osteoarthritis symptoms?

Obesity is a risk factor for OA. It causes increased force across weight-bearing joints, which can contribute to cartilage breakdown and, therefore, to OA. As compared to non-obese people, obese individuals are more likely to develop OA in both knees or in both hips rather than in just one knee or one hip. Interestingly, obesity increases this risk not only for weight-bearing joints such as the knees and hips, but also for non-weight-bearing joints such as the hands. Scientists aren't sure how obesity contributes to OA of the hands, but studies have shown that obese individuals are more likely to develop it.

Body mass index (BMI) is a popular way of evaluating obesity. Your BMI is calculated using a simple formula that takes into account your height in centimeters and your weight in kilograms. Values of about 18.5 to 25 are considered normal; higher numbers indicate overweight or obesity. Having a body mass index in the range of 30–35 increases your risk of developing OA of the knee by four to five times.

If you are overweight, losing weight may help to slow the progression of OA, especially in weight-bearing joints. In addition, weight loss may postpone the need for hip or knee joint replacement. If such surgery is needed, it is likely to have fewer complications in people who are not overweight.

17. Can exercise improve my osteoarthritis symptoms?

Exercise is an excellent therapy for most people with OA. Exercise increases your endurance, muscle strength, and range of motion, and decreases your joint pain. Additionally, it lowers your weight and decreases your risk for high blood pressure, diabetes, and heart disease.

The benefits of exercise in osteoarthritis are especially evident with low-impact, weight-bearing exercises such as walking, biking, swimming, or water aerobics.

The benefits of exercise in OA are especially evident with low-impact, weight-bearing exercises such as walking, biking, swimming, or water aerobics. Exercise equipment such as a treadmill, elliptical glider, or stationary bike can be helpful in this regard as well.

Before beginning any exercise program, you should consult with your doctor. He or she will advise you on the risks associated with the exercise. Your doctor should not only discuss the risks and benefits to your joints, but also include information about other risks associated with exercise, such as those associated with falls or heart attacks.

It makes good sense to start every exercise session with some slow stretching exercises to warm up. A regimen of low-impact exercise that emphasizes increased range of motion is ideal. For example, tai chi or an active range of motion and relaxation program such as "range of motion dance" can help relieve stiffness and improve function. Water exercise is also helpful, especially for people with more advanced arthritis of the hip or knee who would not be able to tolerate conventional exercising in a gym. High-impact exercises such as basketball or volleyball are not a good idea if you have arthritis of the spine, hips, knees, ankles, or feet. The Arthritis Foundation offers exercise classes designed for people with arthritis called PACE (People with Arthritis Can Exercise); contact your local chapter to find out more about these classes.

Mild muscle aches or stiffness after starting an exercise program is normal. If you experience one of these problems, rest for a few days and then try resuming the exercise program at a lower intensity and for a shorter length of time. Over time, you should be able to gradually increase the length of time and the intensity of your exercise program. If exercising leads to severe joint pain, joint swelling, or redness, then you should modify your exercise program. If you are having difficulty finding the right exercise program for use at home or the gym, consult a physical therapist. He or she can help create the most appropriate exercise program for you.

18. Is night pain common in osteoarthritis?

The joint pain associated with OA typically gets worse during exercise and improves with rest. However, when OA is advanced and joints are significantly damaged, patients may experience pain while resting—especially pain at night that keeps them from sleeping. This problem can lead to daytime sleepiness, irritability, clouded thoughts, and depression.

Night pain associated with OA occurs predominantly in the hips and shoulders. It is aggravated by overuse of the joints and improves with several days rest. Individuals who suffer from night pain can benefit from some simple strategies, however.

People with night pain should identify those activities that cause or worsen their night pain, and then avoid or modify these activities so as to reduce the stress on joints. Such modifications might include using a cane when walking, using a motorized wheelchair if walking is too difficult, or using a "grabber" to pick up objects and reduce the amount of back bending necessary.

Use of a firm mattress that distributes the body weight evenly over a large area can also offload pressure on the affected joint. Newer, foam-based mattresses may offer advantages in this regard. Placing pillows between the knees or under the arm may also help to relieve OA-related pain, as may elevating the entire leg with a pillow. You should avoid placing a pillow under the knee so that the knee is flexed for long periods of time, however. Prolonged flexion of the inflamed knee can lead to a contracture of the ligaments and a reduced ability to fully extend the knee. If necessary, you can also try a variety of sleep positions.

If pain persists, taking pain medication before going to sleep may help you to get a good night's rest. Appropriate medications may include nonsteroidal anti-inflammatory drugs (e.g., ibuprofen), narcotic medications (e.g., morphine or hydrocodone), or even antidepressants (e.g., amitriptyline), all of which have been shown to be effective in relieving chronic pain conditions. You should discuss the type and dosage of nighttime medications with your doctor before taking them.

In some cases, night pain caused by OA may be very difficult to endure. Intractable pain may be a sign that it is time to consider surgery.

Night pain caused by osteoarthritis may sometimes be very difficult to endure. Intractable pain may be a sign that it is time to consider surgery.

I experience night pain in my knee and fingers, but not on a regular basis. It seems to happen when I have tried to do too much during the day. Only rarely does it interfere with my sleep.

—George

19. Can osteoarthritis-related foot pain be improved with shoe inserts?

Your foot is a complex structure that includes 26 bones and 33 separate joints. Even in people without OA, foot pain is often difficult to avoid due to the large weight-bearing load placed on the feet. Foot pain in OA is not an unusual symptom. As in the hips, knees, and fingers, OA may affect the cartilage of any or all of the small joints in the feet, resulting in pain and limitation of function. After many years, small fragments of cartilage can come loose and float inside the joints of the foot, which in turn can worsen pain and inflammation. Eventually, the cartilage can erode completely away, so that the bones begin to rub together.

The symptoms of OA of the foot are insidious. They can begin slowly, such that the person experiences minor pain and swelling after extended periods of standing or walking. As the disease progresses and the cartilage wears out, the pain can become intense and seriously impair a person's mobility.

Rheumatologists and orthopedists often suggest that patients with OA of the foot wear sneakers. The insole of a sneaker is made of soft, shock-absorbent material. This kind of padding can cushion the impact associated with walking and help to preserve the knee and foot joints.

Orthotics are devices that fit into shoes and correct foot-related problems. Like sneakers, they can absorb shocks and redistribute pressure so that foot joints are less painful. In-shoe orthotics can be fashioned with a lateral wedge. This wedge, which is made of a firm but flexible material, can help to align the knee joint and take pressure off the medial (inside) portion of the knee joint.

If you have foot or knee pain, in-shoe orthotics may ease your pain and decrease the stress on your joints. Unfortunately, people with diabetes, poor circulation, or swelling can have problems when using orthotics. Your rheumatologist, orthopedist, or podiatrist can evaluate you and determine whether you might benefit from an orthotic.

I am just starting to experience foot pain. It seems to be very bad upon waking and for several minutes after then goes away. Inserts have been recommended but have not tried them yet.

—George

20. What are glucosamine and chondroitin sulfate?

Glucosamine and chondroitin sulfate are both substances that are found naturally in the body. A glucosamine molecule is formed by adding an amino group (NH_2) to a glucose molecule, thereby creating an amino sugar. Glucosamine is a component of a number of structures in the body and is believed to play a role in the formation and repair of cartilage.

Chondroitin sulfate is a member of a class of large molecules called sulfated glycosaminoglycans; these molecules contain sugars, proteins, and sulfur. Chondroitin sulfate is a major constituent in various connective tissues, as well as bone, and cartilage. It is thought to impart elasticity to cartilage.

Both glucosamine and chondroitin sulfate are sold as nutritional supplements. Manufacturers of these supplements extract their raw materials from animal tissue. For example, glucosamine can be extracted from the shells of shrimp, lobsters, or crabs, while chondroitin sulfate can be removed from the cartilage of animals, such as sharks.

21. Do glucosamine and chondroitin sulfate work for osteoarthritis?

Glucosamine and chondroitin sulfate supplements are very popular treatments for OA. Unfortunately, robust scientific evidence that demonstrates their effectiveness in treating this condition is lacking.

Glycosaminoglycans are the building blocks for cartilage. Glucosamine is a precursor to a glycosaminoglycan; chondroitin sulfate is the most common glycosaminoglycan found in human cartilage. The rationale for taking these supplements is the belief that they might help to build new cartilage, repair OA-related damage, or slow the progression of new damage. To date, these purported effects have consisted largely of hopeful speculation, though this speculation has prompted many scientific trials of these supplements.

Unfortunately, the studies performed so far have been of poor quality. Most included only a small number of patients and had a very short duration. Furthermore, many of these studies were underwritten by manufacturers of the supplements (a conflict of interest). Perhaps not surprisingly, the manufacturer-sponsored studies seemed to come up with rosier conclusions than larger, more recent, and more objective studies. As a result, the earlier studies are of limited value when we try to judge the effectiveness of a treatment for a disease that affects millions of people and lasts for many years.

In response to the popularity of these supplements and the lack of good science supporting their use, a branch of the

National Institutes of Health undertook a study to see how these dietary supplements affected OA. This study, which was called the Glucosamine/Chondroitin Arthritis Intervention Trial (GAIT), was the first large-scale, multicenter clinical trial in the United States to test the effects of glucosamine hydrochloride (glucosamine) and sodium chondroitin sulfate (chondroitin sulfate) for treatment of knee OA. The study investigated whether glucosamine and chondroitin sulfate, when used either separately or in combination, reduced pain in patients with knee OA. It reached the following conclusion:

Glucosamine and chondroitin sulfate alone or in combination did not reduce pain *[emphasis added] effectively in the overall group of patients with osteoarthritis of the knee. Exploratory analyses suggest that the combination of glucosamine and chondroitin sulfate* may *[emphasis added] be effective in the subgroup of patients with moderate-to-severe knee pain.*

As discouraging as those results were, many people remain motivated to try these supplements. Patients believe that these supplements are relatively inexpensive and safe. Moreover, many are frustrated with a lack of improvement of their pain from their prescription medications and want to avoid knee replacement surgery.

If you think you might benefit from these supplements or have questions about their risks and benefits, it's worthwhile to discuss this topic with your doctor.

22. Can diacerhein help my osteoarthritis?

Diacerhein is one of the anthraquinones. Anthraquinones are organic compounds derived from plants and animals. They occur naturally in some plants, such as aloe and senna, as well as in fungi, lichens, and insects. Anthraquinones serve as a basic skeleton for these organisms' pigments. Humans have used these substances for centuries for their laxative properties as well as for the production of dyes.

Recently, diacerhein has been used for the treatment of OA by practitioners of alternative medicine. In animal studies, these compounds have been shown to have anti-inflammatory properties as well as a protective effect on cartilage. It is not yet clear whether diacerhein is both safe and effective in humans, however.

Investigators have reviewed seven studies that enrolled people with OA who were treated with diacerhein. These studies included 2069 patients with OA who received diacerhein; these individuals were compared to another group of patients with OA who were treated with a placebo (i.e., sugar pills). When investigators evaluated the group treated with diacerhein, they found that those patients had a statistically significant decrease in pain in the hips and knees. When x-rays of the patients' hips were compared, researchers found a statistically significant slowing of the progression of OA. Evaluations of knee x-rays did not show this benefit. The most frequent adverse event experienced by patients in the diacerhein-treated group was diarrhea.

Overall, for the treatment of OA, these studies demonstrated a small, consistent benefit from taking diacerhein. The long-term effects of taking this compound have not been examined.

23. Is hyaluronic acid an effective treatment for osteoarthritis?

Hyaluronic acid is a clear jelly-like material that is found in many places in the body, including the synovial fluid of joints and the vitreous humor of the eyes. Hyaluronic acid acts as a binding, lubricating, and protective agent and may boost the shock-absorbing properties of a person's joints.

Recognizing hyaluronic acid's many functions in the body, scientists have looked for ways to use it to treat disease. Hyaluronic acid was first used in eye surgery to replace lost vitreous fluids. Today, it is used in plastic surgery to improve the appearance of scars and wrinkles. In this application, Restylane (the brand name for hyaluronic acid) is injected into the skin to "puff up" tissues.

Rheumatologists and orthopedic surgeons have used hyaluronic acid injections to treat the knees of people affected by OA, a type of treatment sometimes called viscosupplementation. The addition of this material to the joints provides a cushioning and lubrication effect. In addition, hyaluronic acid injections provide pain relief even after the medication is no longer detectable in the joint. These injections are an alternative to corticosteroid ("cortisone") injections for people with knee pain that is not manageable with physical therapy and pills.

Hyaluronic acid is not absorbed through the skin, and it cannot be given orally because it is digested by stomach enzymes. Treatment for OA requires a weekly injection into the knee for one to five consecutive weeks, depending on the brand used and based on the doctor's judgment. This type of treatment has several advantages and disadvantages in comparison to cortisone injections. The main advantage is that the pain relief it produces lasts longer than the pain relief offered by a cortisone injection. Treatment can relieve pain for up to 6 months, while cortisone injections provide pain relief for 3–4 weeks only. Studies have shown that treatments can be repeated safely for up to 30 months for the brand Hyalgan. Also, hyaluronic acid does not interfere with other medications you may be taking for osteoarthritis, and is not known to interfere with any other medications. Unfortunately, hyaluronic acid injections may take a little bit longer to work than cortisone injections, and this therapy requires a greater number of visits and injections.

24. I've heard that an antibiotic can help osteoarthritis. Is that true?

It is true that an antibiotic—doxycycline—has been evaluated in the treatment of OA. In studies employing animal models of OA, this drug has been shown to prevent or slow the progression of OA. It is theorized that doxycycline can decrease the amount of cartilage-degrading enzymes found around the joints.

The results in human trials were equivocal, however, and doxycycline had not shown much promise for OA in the past. However, a recently published medical study offers some hope. In this study, obese women with OA-related pain in one knee took 200 milligrams per day of doxycycline for 30 months. Another group of women with similar symptoms were given sugar pills (placebo) to take every day. The patients' pain was assessed at each visit, and x-rays were taken at the beginning and the end of the study. At the end of 30 months, the women who were treated with doxycycline were compared with those who took sugar pills. The results showed that women who took the doxycycline had less pain and less cartilage degradation, as compared to the women who took the sugar pills.

This study is encouraging, but because of several limitations in its design, we cannot say for sure that everyone with OA should start taking doxycycline. For example, the study included only middle-aged women, which begs the question, "Would doxycycline also work in men?" Additionally, the study examined a relatively small number of people (431) and evaluated them over a relatively short period of time. Would the results have been better or worse if the doxycycline therapy was continued? Experts have suggested that before doxycycline can be recommended as a treatment, larger studies must be done. The populations of the studies should include men and women as well as people from a variety of ethnic backgrounds. Until this kind of research is carried out, doxycycline should not be routinely prescribed for people with OA.

25. Can my osteoarthritis symptoms be improved with surgery?

Many surgical interventions can provide relief of OA-related symptoms. They range from office procedures that your rheumatologist can do under local anesthesia to major surgery performed by orthopedic surgery specialists that requires you to be hospitalized. These procedures include the injection of hyaluronic acid, steroids, or even new cartilage cells (chondrocytes) into the joint; arthroscopic procedures; and total joint replacement. The type of procedure that you might need depends on many factors, including your symptoms, the amount of disability you have, your general health status, and the skills and training of your orthopedic surgeon.

If you have OA of any joint that has progressed to the point it limits your ability to function or enjoy life, then you should consider surgery. For example, if you have hip or knee pain that cannot be controlled with medication or if your joint is so degenerated by OA that it no longer functions, then surgery may offer significant relief of pain and improvement in function.

The ultimate outcome of most orthopedic surgery depends on two factors: the skills of the surgeon and the willingness and ability of the patient to participate in a rehabilitation program for weeks or months after the procedure.

Unlike other types of surgery (for example, having your appendix removed), orthopedic surgery requires a greater investment of your time and effort after the procedure. The ultimate outcome of most orthopedic surgery depends on two factors: the skills of the surgeon and the willingness and ability of the patient to participate in a rehabilitation program for weeks or months after the procedure. Patients without the physical or mental ability to participate in a rigorous rehabilitation program are not considered good candidates for many procedures.

If you are considering surgery, discuss this issue with your primary care physician and your rheumatologist. They can advise you if you are a good candidate for a surgical procedure and explain what you can expect after the surgery.

26. Will my knee feel better if the doctor removes the fluid in it?

OA of the knees sometimes causes fluid to fill the joint, which causes swelling and pain. While this condition is commonly called "water on the knee," doctors may refer to the increased fluid more formally as a joint effusion. All of the movable (diarthrodial) joints in the body are surrounded by a layer of cells called the synovial membrane. This layer of cells normally produces a small amount of fluid, whose purpose is to lubricate the joints. OA can lead to irritation of the synovium and cause it to produce larger than normal amounts of joint fluid. This extra fluid may create visible swelling of the knee as well as increased pain and stiffness. If you develop swelling and pain in your knee, your doctor may suggest that you have the fluid removed in a procedure called an **arthrocentesis.**

Arthrocentesis

The removal of fluid from a joint; also called joint aspiration. In this procedure, a sterile needle and syringe are used to drain fluid from a joint that is inflamed or infected.

Your physician may remove this fluid for two reasons. First, the procedure is diagnostic and can help your doctor determine what is causing the swelling. Second, the procedure itself may be therapeutic and help relieve the pain and stiffness of the knee.

The symptoms of swelling, pain, and stiffness in the knee can also be caused by processes other than OA, the most dangerous of which is an infection of the joint. If your doctor is not sure what is causing your knee pain and swelling, removing the joint fluid from the knee can help him or her to make a diagnosis of OA and exclude more serious problems such as joint infection (septic arthritis). Examination of the physical properties of the joint fluid, such as its color and clarity, and its white blood cell count can assist the physician in making these important determinations.

The removal of excess joint fluid can relieve pain, swelling, and stiffness, and improve the knee's range of motion and flexibility. Additionally, chronic knee effusions sometimes contribute to leg weakness. Removing extra joint fluid can be helpful in rebuilding quadriceps strength as well. The doctor may also inject corticosteroids ("cortisone") into the knee in an attempt to relieve arthritis symptoms. Sometimes this type of injection helps to prevent the joint fluid from reaccumulating. Corticosteroids can be injected approximately every three months, but if necessary the knee joint fluid can be drained more frequently.

Before performing an arthrocentesis, your doctor will clean your knee and the surrounding area with an antiseptic soap. Next, the doctor will inject a medication, such as lidocaine, into the skin to numb the area. Finally, he or she will use a hypodermic needle to draw off the fluid. In experienced hands, this procedure does not cause much discomfort and usually takes five to ten minutes. You do not need to do any special preparation before this procedure, and you will usually feel better immediately.

27. Will arthroscopy help the pain in my knees?

Arthroscopy is a form of minimally invasive surgery that is performed on joints that have been injured through accident or disease. Arthroscopic procedures can be performed without opening the joint. These types of procedures have a lower risk of surgical complications than more invasive surgeries, reduce the amount of time you must spend in the hospital, and are associated with a quicker return to normal activity.

In arthroscopy, a specially trained surgeon passes a tube, known as an arthroscope, into the joint. The arthroscope contains both a light and a camera. It allows the surgeon to visualize structures inside the joint through a very small hole in the skin. Using another small hole, the surgeon can insert surgical instruments into the joint to repair injured structures. Sometimes a third incision is made so that the surgeon can insert additional surgical instruments or remove pieces of cartilage or bone that are causing pain and inflammation.

More than 500,000 arthroscopic procedures are performed each year in the United States. Approximately half of those patients report an improvement in pain and function after undergoing this type of surgery. The most common joint that arthroscopy is used on is the knee, and the most commonly performed arthroscopic procedures are tidal lavage and chondroplasty.

In **tidal lavage,** the surgeon removes small pieces of cartilage and other debris from the inside of the joint. After anesthetizing the patient, the surgeon injects sterile salt water into the joint several times. This fluid is allowed to wash out of another small hole in the joint. Many patients experience decreased pain and increased function following this procedure, with the improvements lasting several weeks or months.

Tidal lavage

A treatment for osteoarthritis of the knee in which a saline solution is repeatedly injected, then withdrawn from the joint space to remove debris from the joint and help break up the synovial membrane, which has adhered to itself.

In chondroplasty, the surgeon removes damaged cartilage from the joint and replaces it with new cartilage. The surgeon shaves off damaged cartilage from the inside of the joint and then removes some healthy cartilage from a part of the joint that does not bear weight or come in contact with other bones. The healthy cartilage is sent to a laboratory, which removes the healthy cartilage cells (called chondrocytes) from the cartilage. These new chondrocytes are placed back in the joint during a second surgical procedure. Some patients experience improvement in pain and function in their joints after this procedure. Chondroplasty is currently recommended for younger patients with joint injuries who want to prevent OA by repairing defective joint surfaces.

A study conducted in 2002 examined the effectiveness of arthroscopy in patients with OA of the knees. In half of the patients, an actual arthroscopic procedure was performed. In the other half, incisions were made in the skin of the knees of the anesthetized patients to make them think they had undergone surgery. When the physicians examined the patients and followed their progress over two years, they discovered that arthroscopic knee surgery was no more effective than sham surgery for relief of pain or stiffness from OA.

While this study doesn't mean that arthroscopy does not offer any benefit to any patient, its results should prompt debate on which procedure to perform and who is most likely to benefit. If you are considering arthroscopic surgery, discuss the likely risks and benefits with your rheumatologist and your orthopedist. Acting collaboratively, you should decide whether you are the best candidate for this procedure.

28. Is joint replacement an option for the treatment of osteoarthritis symptoms?

Currently, medical science provides no cure for OA. Nevertheless, many therapies can reduce OA-related pain and increase joint function, including anti-inflammatory agents, painkillers, physical therapy, braces, orthotics, and lifestyle changes. All of these measures have been shown to reduce the symptoms of the disease. However, when these conservative treatments no longer provide relief, surgery is an option. This includes joint replacement surgery.

When conservative treatments for osteoarthritis no longer provide relief, surgery—including joint replacement—is an option.

The replacement of a natural joint with an artificial joint (i.e., prosthesis) is carried out through a surgical procedure called an arthroplasty. The two most commonly performed joint replacement procedures are hip and knee arthroplasties. Both are very successful procedures and are associated with high rates of patient satisfaction. They are by no means the only joint replacement procedures, however: Shoulder, elbow, wrist, and finger joints can also be replaced.

Not every person with an arthritic joint is a candidate for joint replacement. Joint replacement surgery is indicated for people who are in pain and have significant limitations of movement in the affected joint. These patients have usually failed to respond the more conservative treatment options. Even if a person meets all of these criteria, however, surgery may not be the most appropriate option. If the patient has other conditions that would increase the risk of complications or of prosthetic failure or that would render the individual unable to participate in a rigorous rehabilitation program, then he or she is unlikely to be considered for this type of surgery. For example, people with severe neurological, intellectual, or psychiatric impairment would not be able to participate in rehabilitation, nor would patients with severe heart or lung conditions. People with severe osteoporosis or obesity would also be at high risk for a failure of the prosthesis. Those with blood clotting disorders could be at excessive risk of pulmonary embolism (blood clots in the lung), strokes, or bleeding after surgery.

The timing of the surgery is important. For example, studies suggest that if a joint replacement is delayed too long, patients may become too debilitated to participate in their physical therapy after surgery. If a young person needs a joint replacement, his or her orthopedist will delay this surgery for as long as possible, because the implanted prosthesis will wear out. Thus a younger patient may eventually require one or more additional replacements in the future. Ideally, as surgical techniques and materials science improve over time, newer prostheses will be more durable and will require fewer replacements.

29. Can acupuncture improve my osteoarthritis-related pain?

Acupuncture is a branch of traditional Chinese medicine. It is based on the premise that the healthy body circulates an energy known as qi or chi. This energy circulates between the vital organs along channels or meridians. Blockages in these meridians result in an imbalance of qi, which results in disease. The traditional acupuncturist seeks to find the source of the imbalance and correct it by applying needles to various points along the meridians, called acupoints. More modern acupuncturists may employ other modalities to "unblock" the meridians, such as electricity, heat, pressure, and even laser light.

Numerous studies have examined the use of acupuncture in patients with OA. Recently, scientists at the U.S. National Health Service (NHS), a part of the U.S. Department of Health and Human Services, reviewed all of the available studies on the use of acupuncture for the treatment of OA. These researchers noted that the results of these studies were often confounded by small patient populations, variations in acupuncture technique, and the difficulty associated with finding an adequate "placebo" or sham procedure with which to compare the acupuncture. Nevertheless, they noted that most of these studies did not find a benefit for acupuncture when compared to sham acupuncture. They concluded that while the evidence is not sufficient to justify acupuncture as first-line treatment, it was probably sufficient to justify its use as a second- or third-line treatment. In addition, the authors suggested that the most appropriate candidate for acupuncture was a person who was not responding to conventional management, not tolerating medication, or experiencing recurrent pain.

Acupuncture is not without its downside. It is associated with some serious adverse events, including transmission of infectious disease, lung puncture (pneumothorax), other problems associated with organ punctures, spinal injuries, bleeding around the heart (cardiac tamponade), and broken needles left in the skin or other organs. Minor adverse events can include needles forgotten by the acupuncturist, worsening of pain and stiffness, minor bleeding, bruising, fatigue, sweating, severe nausea, fainting, and headache. The risk of adverse events tends to vary based on the practitioner's level of competence and training.

30. Is water therapy effective in the treatment of osteoarthritis-related pain and stiffness?

Water therapy, also known as pool therapy, aqua therapy, or hydrotherapy, can be effective in reducing the symptoms of OA. In particular, it can be a soothing way to stretch your muscles and reduce the pain from the impact of exercise done on land.

A heated pool is a great environment for exercise. It major advantage over land-based exercise is the heat and buoyancy provided by the water.

The heat of a warmed pool relaxes tired muscles and reduces aches and pains, which in turn allows for longer and less painful exercise sessions. The ideal temperature for water exercises is 83 to 88 degrees Fahrenheit. If the water is cooler, it does not relax the muscles as well. If the water temperature is higher, you can easily overheat while exercising.

Buoyancy is the tendency for a body to float in a liquid. It counteracts the press of gravity. For example, if you stand up to your neck in water, your feet support only 10% of your body weight; the water supports the rest. Someone standing up to his waist in water supports only 50% of his body weight. Reduced weight bearing reduces the stress across the joints, which in turn reduces the pain associated with OA and allows for longer and more vigorous exercise. This type of exercise is particularly helpful to patients with OA in the spine, hips, and knees, for whom almost any other exercise is too painful to tolerate.

Pools are not just for swimming, of course. Numerous forms of exercises can be practiced in the pool. Unlike similar exercises performed on land, exercises in the pool take advantage of both the buoyancy and the gentle resistance of the water against arms and legs. Types of exercises practiced in pools include the following:

- *Water aerobics*—including calisthenics, running in place, water walking, or using cross-country skiing movements in a shallow pool.
- *Stretching*—including stretching the lower back, hamstrings, and calf muscles; touching the toes; and slowly raising the knees to the chest.
- *Strengthening*—including muscle-building exercises, the use of foam barbells or hand paddles to complete bicep curls, and lateral side raises that work against water resistance.
- *Ai chi*—a form of tai chi that was developed specifically for exercise in pools. Its slow, gentle, and rhythmic movements develop strength, balance, and joint flexibility.

As with any exercise program, you should start by visiting your doctor and making sure that you can tolerate the exercise without undue risk before you begin any type of water therapy.

31. Can cartilage be replaced?

Surgery for the repair of knee cartilage is commonplace today. It involves removing loose cartilage and smoothing the surface of existing cartilage. But what if cartilage is missing—can a defect in the surface of the cartilage be repaired in such a case? In fact, surgeons in Sweden began performing this type of surgery more than a decade ago. They removed small, matchstick-shaped pieces of cartilage from areas of the knee that did not bear weight and inserted them into areas on the weight-bearing surface where cartilage was missing. This technique worked reasonably well—but what if you did not have enough cartilage tissue to graft?

To address this issue, scientists developed a process for harvesting cartilage cells, growing them outside the body, and then replacing them into a damaged joint. The company that initially developed this laboratory technique, Genzyme Biosurgery, calls its product Carticel. More generally, the surgical procedure of harvesting, culturing, and replacing the cells is called autologous chondrocyte implantation (ACI) or autologous chondrocyte transfer (ACT). The word "autologous" means that the person uses his or her own cartilage cells to grow new cells; that is, the cells are not donated by another person.

The ACI technique involves a two-step surgical procedure. In the first surgery, the surgeon removes a small amount of cartilage tissue. The cells in this tissue (chondrocytes) are then brought to a lab, where they can be grown and the population of cells can be multiplied. When there are a sufficient number of cells (usually after a few weeks), a second surgery is performed, in which the cells are placed in the cartilage defect in the joint. Over time, these cells develop into cartilage and significantly improve the function of the joint.

The disadvantages of this procedure include its high cost and the length of the rehabilitation following the surgery, which can take months of exercise and crutch walking. This technique has been approved by the FDA for people who have experienced cartilage-related injuries from sports or other accidents, but it is not an approved therapy for people with OA.

Research continues on ways to employ ACI to help patients with OA. For example, tissue engineers are working on techniques to grow larger amounts of chondrocytes in a customized mold that has the same size and shape as the damaged joint surface. It is hoped that these cells will be able to replace all of the cartilage in a joint and that their implantation will not require the prolonged rehabilitation period needed today.

32. What are other resources for people with osteoarthritis?

The following websites, books, and magazines may be helpful to patients with osteoarthritis.

Organizations

American College of Rheumatology
1800 Century Place
Suite 250
Atlanta, GA 30345-4300
Phone: 404-633-3777
Fax: 404-633-1870
http://www.rheumatology.org
The American College of Rheumatology is an organization of and for physicians, health professionals, and scientists. Its goal is to advance rheumatology through programs of education, research, advocacy, and practice support that foster excellence in the care of people with arthritis and rheumatic and musculoskeletal diseases.

Arthritis Foundation
P.O. Box 7669
Atlanta, GA 30357-0669
Phone: 800-568-4045
http://www.arthritis.org
Currently this website has a link with which you can obtain a free kit on rheumatoid arthritis. "It is designed to give you tools and tips to better communicate with your rheumatologist about your symptoms and how to get the most from your office visits." The Arthritis Foundation provides lots of information on arthritis, and a long list of useful links to other websites.

Arthritis National Research Foundation
200 Oceangate
Suite 830
Long Beach, CA 90802

Phone: 800-588-2873
Fax: 562-983-1410
E-mail: anrf@ix.netcom.com
The Arthritis National Research Foundation offers funding to promising young scientists at the beginning of their research careers to pursue cutting-edge projects for the treatment, cure, and eventual end to the suffering of the more than 66 million Americans with arthritis and its related diseases.

Arthritis Research Institute of America
300 South Duncan Avenue
Suite 188
Clearwater, FL 33755
Phone: 727-461-4054
Fax: 727-449-9227
E-mail: info@preventarthritis.org
The Arthritis Research Institute of America is a national nonprofit, public charity with tax-exempt status. The institute was founded on the premise that important areas of arthritis research needed to be addressed, that the urgency of those needs was increasing, and that the institute could provide effective, innovative, and cost-effective ways to meet those needs. The institute's mission is to identify the causes, seek preventive measures, and find a cure for osteoarthritis. The nature of the research is primarily community-based studies as well as clinical studies.

Arthritis Society (National Office)
393 University Avenue, Suite 1700
Toronto, Ontario M5G 1E6
Canada
Phone: 416-979-7228
Fax: 416-979-8366
E-mail: info@arthritis.ca

Websites

Johns Hopkins Arthritis Center
www.hopkins-arthritis.som.jhmi.edu/index.html
The Johns Hopkins Arthritis Center is a very useful source of scientific updates in the field of arthritis. Its website is a great resource for both doctors and patients. The site includes an entire section on rheumatoid arthritis. You can also download a rheumatoid arthritis activity minder—a tool for monitoring disease activity so you can objectively keep track of your course and have better communication with your doctor.

MayoClinic.com
http://www.mayoclinic.com/health/rheumatoid-arthritis/DS00020/DSECTION=8&
This is a great website from the people at the Mayo Clinic. It has excellent information about rheumatoid arthritis and its treatments.

Medicinenet
http://www.medicinenet.com/rheumatoid_arthritis/article.htm
MedicineNet.com is an online, healthcare media publishing company. Its website provides authoritative medical information on rheumatoid arthritis and other topics for consumers.

Medline Plus
www.nlm.nih.gov/medlineplus/medlineplus.html
Medline plus is a project of the National Library of Medicine. This website provides useful information on almost any topic and includes very useful information on medications.

Magazines

Arthritis Today
This magazine, which is available from the Arthritis Foun-

dation, contains useful articles on how to live with rheumatoid arthritis and updates medications and new treatments.

Audacity Magazine
This news and entertainment magazine is geared toward the disability community in the United States and the world.

Books

The Arthritis Helpbook
By Kate Lorig and James Fries
Available from the Arthritis Foundation or from booksellers. This is a very helpful book with useful tips for learning to live with arthritis.

Glossary

A

Arthr-: A prefix meaning "joint."

Arthritis: Inflammation of a joint, usually accompanied by pain, swelling, and stiffness.

Arthrocentesis: The removal of fluid from a joint; also called joint aspiration. In this procedure, a sterile needle and syringe are used to drain fluid from a joint that is inflamed or infected.

Arthroplasty: Implantation of a mechanical joint to replace a diseased or damaged joint; also called total joint replacement surgery.

Arthroscopy: A diagnostic and surgical technique that uses a thin tube with a light and a tiny video camera at one end to view the inside of a joint.

Articular cartilage: Tough, rubbery tissue that forms the surface of bones within joints.

B

Bisphosphonate: One of a class of drugs used to maintain or improve bone density.

Bone remodeling: A cyclical process by which bone maintains a dynamic steady state through resorption and formation of a small amount of bone at the same site. Bone remodeling can occur as a result of joint disease.

Bouchard's nodes: Knobby overgrowths of the middle joint of the fingers in people with osteoarthritis.

C

Chondrocyte: A cartilage cell.

Chondroitin sulfate: A sugar-based material that is present in cartilage. Chondroitin is a popular dietary supplement that is thought to improve the joint symptoms of osteoarthritis.

Chronic: Lasting for a long time. The word comes from the Greek *chronos,* which means "time."

Collagen: The major protein of connective tissue, cartilage, and bone.

Connective tissue: The material that holds various body structures together. Cartilage, tendons, ligaments, and blood vessels are composed entirely of connective tissue.

Coronary artery disease: A narrowing of the coronary arteries that results in inadequate blood flow to the heart.

Corticosteroids: Any of the steroid hormones made by the cortex (outer layer) of the adrenal gland; also called cortisol and steroids. These potent drugs are used to reduce the pain and inflammation associated with rheumatoid arthritis and other autoimmune disorders.

D

Degenerative joint disease (DJD): Joint destruction that occurs over a long period of time. This term is used synonymously with the term "osteoarthritis."

Diagnosis: The identification of an illness after review of the patient's clinical history, physical exam, and laboratory tests.

E

Enzyme: Any protein that regulates chemical changes in other substances.

Erosion: From the Latin *erodere,* meaning "to eat away"; an eating away of a surface. Erosion of the bone surface of joints is a common feature of many types of arthritis.

F

Fatigue: A condition characterized by a lessened capacity for work and reduced efficiency of accomplishment, usually accompanied by a feeling of weariness and tiredness.

Flare: The reappearance or worsening of arthritic symptoms.

G

Glucosamine: An amino sugar produced by the body that is found in cartilage. Glucosamine is a popular dietary supplement and is thought to improve the joints symptoms of osteoarthritis.

Gout: A disease characterized by increased blood levels of uric acid; it produces pain and inflammation in the joints, particularly in the foot, ankle, and knee.

H

Heberden's nodes: Knobby overgrowths of the joint nearest the fingertips in patients with osteoarthritis.

I

Inflammation: A response to injury or foreign invasion that is designed to protect the body. Its symptoms include heat, redness, swelling, and pain.

L

Ligament: A thin layer of connective tissue that holds the tooth in its socket, and acts as a cushion between tooth and bone.

M

Magnetic resonance imaging (MRI): A diagnostic technique in which radio waves generated in a strong magnetic field are used to provide information about the hydrogen atoms in different tissues within the body. A computer then uses this information to produce images of the tissues in many different planes.

N

Nonsteroidal anti-inflammatory drugs (NSAIDs): Medications that relieve joint pain and stiffness by reducing inflammation. Examples include aspirin and ibuprofen.

O

Osteoarthritis (OA): A type of arthritis characterized by pain and stiffness in the joints, such as those in the hands, hips, knees, spine, or feet; it is caused by the breakdown of cartilage.

Osteophyte: An outgrowth of bone.

Osteoporosis: A disease characterized by the thinning of the bones with a reduction in bone mass owing to depletion of calcium and bone protein. Osteoporosis predisposes a person to fractures.

P

Primary osteoarthritis: The gradual breakdown of cartilage that occurs with age and is caused by stress on a joint.

Progressive: An adjective applied to many diseases; it suggests an increase in scope or severity of disease.

R

Range of motion (ROM): Measurement of joint movement angle, which may be restricted due to inflammation.

Rheumatoid arthritis (RA): A chronic autoimmune disease characterized by pain, stiffness, inflammation, swelling, and sometimes destruction of joints.

Rheumatologist: A physician who specializes in the treatment of diseases of the joints and connective tissue.

Rheumatology: The branch of medicine devoted to the study and treatment of connective tissue diseases.

S

Secondary osteoarthritis: Osteoarthritis that results from trauma to the joint or from chronic joint injury due to another type of arthritis, such as rheumatoid arthritis.

Septic arthritis: Arthritis caused by invading microorganisms.

Side effects: A term associated with medical treatments; problems that occur when a treatment has consequences that go beyond the desired effect, or when the patient develops problems that occur in addition to the desired therapeutic effect.

Synovial fluid: A lubricating fluid secreted by the synovial membrane.

Synovial membrane: Connective tissue that lines the cavity of a joint and produces synovial fluid.

Synovitis: Inflammation of the synovium.

T

Tidal lavage: A treatment for osteoarthritis of the knee in which a saline solution is repeatedly injected, then withdrawn from the joint space to remove debris from the joint and help break up the synovial membrane, which has adhered to itself.

Total hip replacement: A type of surgery in which the diseased ball and socket of the hip joint are completely removed and replaced with artificial materials. Also called a hip arthroplasty.

Total knee replacement: A surgical procedure in which damaged parts of the knee joint are replaced with artificial parts, which are usually made of plastic and steel.

V

Viscosupplementation: A treatment option for people with osteoarthritis of the knee that involves the injection of hyaluronan, a natural component of synovial fluid, directly into the knee joint.

Vitamin D: A fat-soluble vitamin that causes the intestines to increase absorption and metabolism of the minerals calcium and phosphorus (the building blocks of bone).

Index